Ketogenic Diet Rapid Weight Loss Dinners:

Lose Up To 30 LBS. In 30 Days

Henry Brooke

Table of Contents

Introduction

Want to lose 30 pounds in 30 days?

YOU CAN with the metabolism boosting Ketogenic Diet Plan!

Crash dieting is something pretty much everyone on the planet has tried at one time or another.

NEWSFLASH - It doesn't work!

Livestrong experts report up to 65% of dieters return to their pre-dieting weight before the 3 year mark. That's according to *Gary Foster, Ph.D.*, Director of the Eating Disorder Program at the University of Pennsylvania.

The Ketogenic Diet can be used for successful rapid weight loss when used properly. And THOUSANDS of people report up to a pound a day lost!

This is an introductory take-action guide for understanding and using the Ketogenic Diet to lose weight fast and effectively. It will give you a huge advantage in forcing your body to lose fat and keep it off for life!

Nutrition and fitness professionals around the globe recommend healthy dietary changes and regular exercise to lose weight permanently. This is where the Ketogenic Diet comes in. An eating strategy that's not about starving yourself. It's a scientifically proven diet to lose weight that actually forces your body to chemically alter the fuel your body normally uses for energy. With the Ketogenic low-carb eating style you force your body to maximize fat burn for energy and blast fat stores in the process.

Is the Ketogenic Diet safe?

The American Journal of Clinical Nutrition points out no species could have survived millions of years without natural periods where glucose wasn't available for energy burn. Scientists also point out that natural ketogenesis occurs when you are sleeping.

And because of the high-fat intake the Ketogenic Diet allows calories to be cut drastically without feeling deprived and hungry.

There are thousands of people eating Ketogenic style that have claimed to lose between 20 and 30 pounds in just one month! *The Ketogenic Diet Resource* has success stories with people happily losing 30 pounds in 30 days and going strong!

We are going to have a look at the Ketogenic Diet for weight loss and other natural health benefits, while outlining a sample eating plan, food list, and exercise tips to help you reach your weight loss goals quickly. **FAST** weight loss is the focus and this eating strategy can make it happen for **YOU**.

This guide teaches you all about the Ketogenic Diet basics and how you can use this fast weight loss eating plan to rejig your body to use fat stores for energy first, while guiding you step by step towards a healthier lifestyle.

Don't miss out on this guide that teaches you how to take control of your fat TODAY!

The Ketogenic Diet was created or developed in the 20th century to successfully treat young children suffering from epileptic seizures. It also shows promise with controlling weight and blood sugars in diabetics, and incredibly fast weight loss. I hope 30 pounds in 30 days works for you!

So how exactly does this diet work?

This Ketogenic Diet is an all-natural high-fat, moderate protein, low-carb diet that was initially created for medicinal purposes but has recently taken the world by storm because it triggers **FAST** weight loss.

In basic this diet switches things up by forcing the body to ditch the glucose usually used for energy and burn fat. Most people eat plenty of carbohydrates that are broken down into glucose and used for energy, particularly in brain and nervous system function.

When you systematically remove most of the carbohydrate foods from your diet the liver has no choice but to transform fat into fatty acids and ketone bodies. Now these ketones migrate into your brain for energy use instead of glucose. Looking at the medical end of it, a higher level of ketones in the blood reduces the frequency of seizures.

And for the rest of us, there's nothing wrong with burning fat, right?

Main Benefits of the Ketogenic Diet

Authoritynutrition.com recommends you have your blood work done before you start the Ketogenic Diet so you can measure your progress after you've been on the diet a few months.

Banishes Sugar Cravings - By having a solid healthy supply of nutrients in your system void of unhealthy simple sugars, your usual roller coaster of high and low energy levels will disappear, along with sugar cravings.

Decrease Hunger - _eatingacademy.com_ reports ketone bodies take a big bite out of your appetite, and fat makes you feel full longer. Feeling satiated with healthy food is a HUGE benefit when losing weight.

Improved Digestion and Faster Healing - Carbohydrates are associated with inflammation, bloating, gas, and stomach pain. Removing them with Ketogenic eating reduces these annoying symptoms.

Levels Mood - Studies show ketone bodies help stabilize the nervous system which settles dopamine and serotonin levels and puts you in good spirits.

Increased Energy - Healthy protein and good fat provide great long-term clean energy. You will notice quality energy with this diet.

Weight Loss - For normal metabolic function the Ketogenic Diet is excellent for fast weight loss. Drastically reducing your carbohydrate intake reduces glucose availability and forces a chemical change where your body uses fat for energy instead of glucose. And by throwing in a routine exercise program you will intensify your results and look and feel like a million bucks!

Risks of Low-Carb, High-Protein Diet

Kidney Issues - If you have kidney problems you can strain your kidneys further by eating too much protein according to experts at *WebMD*. So check with your doctor before starting.

Future Osteoporosis - Studies show some people have a tendency to pee out more calcium than normal if eating lots of protein. This is something else to talk to your medical provider about.

Elevated Cholesterol/Increased Risk of Cardiovascular Disease - If you are eating unhealthy fatty meat protein in large quantities and full fat dairy in the extreme, you are at risk for increasing you cholesterol level and boosting your risk of heart disease. This is where you need to get smart about what you're eating and take into consideration your risk factors; lifestyle, goals, age, and genetic predisposition. Your doctor can help you with all of that.

HUGE MISCONCEPTION

You may have heard that ketosis is dangerous. You need to understand the difference between **Diabetic Ketoacidosis** and **Nutritional Ketosis.** Here's a little of the basics to help you understand. Your body produces three ketone bodies from fat and amino acids and manufactures ketones for survival.

FACT - Your brain only functions on glucose and ketones. And science says you can't store glucose for more than 24 hours, which means you'd die of hypoglycemia if you were forced to fast more than 24 hours and had no ketones. Luckily your liver can use amino acids and fat to make ketones to appease your brain's hunger.

Diabetic Ketoacidosis (DKA) is when a diabetic doesn't get enough insulin and literally goes into starvation mode. Sure they may have plenty of glucose available in their bloodstream but if they don't have the insulin to make it useable their cells and brain won't get it.

Naturally in defense the body makes ketones from fat. This would normally be a good thing but in a diabetic it isn't because there isn't a feedback loop to regulate this production or turn it off, and the body will just keep on making ketones from fat and amino acids for energy. Eventually this process will cause serious issues with the metabolic derangement of the patient and make them very ill. Ketones are essential but if they aren't regulated they will become toxic in diabetics.

This serious state is not possible in the average person even if they only produce small amounts of insulin. The feedback loop is created and the ketone production is regulated and safe. Yes it's safe to use **Nutritional Ketosis** (Ketogenic Diet) for fast weight loss. This is where the brain shifts and uses fat for energy instead of glucose, with the result of quick fat loss. A healthy individual losing fat with the Ketogenic Diet has no chance of experiencing DKA.

These two types of ketosis have about as much in common as a mud-puddle and the ocean. Now let's have a look at what you should and shouldn't be eating!

It's important to have the take-action information available to understand how to lose weight fast. So we're going to get down to business with an easy to follow food list for you to ensure you keep your pantry, fridge, and freezer stocked with Ketogenic Diet-friendly foods!

This diet is about eating **REAL** food. Look to stick with lean meat, eggs, yogurt, veggies, and sometimes fruit. Processed foods aren't on your list so steer clear of them!

GO FOR IT FOODS

Preferred Wild Free Range Animals Grass Fed (2-3 servings per day)

Pork - Ham, pork tenderloin, and pork chops (watch out for hidden sugars).

Whole Eggs - Free range is preferred and you can have them hard boil, fried, poached, scrambled, or deviled.

Fresh or Frozen Fish - Wild fish is best so you know it's free of any harmful chemicals or additives. Great choices are salmon, tuna, halibut, snapper, trout, and mackerel.

Meat - Grass fed is best and great options are beef, lamb, veal, goat, bison, and other game.

Shellfish - Lobster, shrimp, oysters, crab, squid, mussels, and scallops work.

Poultry - You want free range if possible and chicken, turkey, pheasant, and quail are great.

Peanut Butter - Natural nut butters are great. Be careful there aren't extra carbohydrates and sugar added.

Bacon/Sausage - Be very careful they don't contain fillers and aren't cured with sugar.

Good Healthy Fats (5-7 servings per day)

Note: Fats are a large part of the Ketogenic Diet and you want to make sure you get your Omega Fatty Acids by having 2-3 servings of fatty fish each week. If not, you should take a fish oil supplement just to be safe!

*Avocado, butter, ghee, and beef tallow

*Chicken fat, macadamia nuts, lard (non-hydrogenated), and mayonnaise

*Peanut butter, nut butter, and olive oil

*Coconut oil, red palm oil, and coconut butter

Veggies Minus The Starch (6-10 servings per day)

Note: Go for the low-carb green leafy veggies first. Choose higher carb options like shallots, carrots, snow peas, and green beans less often. You really can't knock yourself out of ketosis if you are choosing non-starch low-carb vegetables.

*Lettuce, spinach, chard, and chives
*Bok choy, bamboo shoots, celery, and radishes
*Seaweed, kale, mushrooms, cabbage, and avocado
*Avocado, okra, asparagus, fennel, and cucumbers
*Broccoli, cauliflower, peppers, Brussels sprouts, and squash
*Zucchini, tomatoes, artichokes, eggplant, and turnip
*Pumpkin, leeks, water chestnuts, and rutabagas

Dairy Foods (2-3 servings per day)

When possible full-fat and free-range are what you're looking for with the Ketogenic Diet.

*Full-fat whipping cream, sour cream, and cottage cheese
*Both hard and soft cheeses (feta, Swiss, cheddar, mozzarella, Monterey Jack, and Colby)
*Milk and yogurt

Seeds and Nuts (2-3 servings per day)

Note: Roasting nuts is best to remove any impurities and peanuts aren't really recommended, as they are a legume anyway.

*Macadamias, almonds, and walnuts are the best low-carb options.
*Pistachios and cashews are allowed in moderation because they are higher in carbs.

Note: Baking with nut and seed flours is okay in moderation.

Drinks

Your best choice is always water and you should be gulping at least 6-8 glasses per day. Clear soups also count along with herbal tea. Many people want to know if they can drink alcohol on this diet. The best answer is **NO** because they are loaded with sugars. However some people find balance with a lower carb option like vodka on occasion. Studies from *the ketogenicdiet.org* state people that tried to slip wine in ended up predominantly stalling weight loss efforts.

Moderation is key and if you happen to have a drink on the odd special occasion it's not going to kill you. Just don't make a habit of it.

No-Kay Foods on the Ketogenic Diet

Foods favored with this diet are typically high-fat, moderate protein, and low-carb. So a great example would be a spinach salad with grilled chicken, olives, avocado, tomatoes, peppers, Swiss cheese, and drizzled with coconut oil dressing. So it makes sense to avoid foods that are high-carb, low-fat. Make sure you aren't eating a giant plate of pasta for dinner or scarfing down muffins, pastries, or no-fat cookies for your snacks!

No Sugar or Diet Soda

You might think diet soda is okay for you because it doesn't have carbs or sugars. In theory yes, but experts at prevention.com remind us it's the artificial sweeteners that are the problem. Everyone reacts differently to them and the last thing you want is to work hard to lose weight quickly and have this oversight block your weight loss success.

Packaged, Shelf, and Processed Foods

Sweet and trans-fat loaded processed foods are filled with high carbs, and additives and preservatives that are nasty for your system. Processed, boxed, and packaged foods are usually full of sugar and all sorts of unhealthy ingredients you probably can't even pronounce.

Skip the fast food processed foods and opt for all-natural and wholesome when you're looking to lose weight **FAST** on the Ketogenic Diet.

Low-Carb Snacks and Sweets

Just because these treats are advertised low-carb doesn't mean they are. Many still contain processed food and lots of carbs. It all adds up so be careful.

Fruit

It's no secret fruits are full of carbohydrates. Which means you should avoid them for the most part. Even though fruits have natural sugars they are sugars nonetheless. In general try and stay away from high carb fruits like bananas, grapes, peaches, nectarines, strawberries, grapes, apricots, watermelon, strawberry, raspberries, cranberries, and blueberries. Find your balance and if you need to slip some berries in with your morning yogurt it's not the end of the world.

This includes fruit juices too.

Grains

These should be avoided completely. Breads, cakes, pastries, cookies, and foods made from flour shouldn't be on the menu. Breadcrumbs and rice should also be avoided.

Veggies Underground

Health experts from *Women's Day* report most vegetables that grow beneath the earth's surface have higher levels of carbs. Veggies like carrots, potatoes, and onions should be avoided when possible on the Ketogenic Diet.

Now that you've got the basics for what foods fit and don't fit so well with this fat burning eating strategy, let's move onto your sample meal plan.

Salads

Keto fast salad

Serves: 2

Time: 20 minutes

Ingredients:

- 4oz. ham
- 1oz. blue cheese
- 2 eggs, hard-boiled
- ½ avocado, sliced
- 4 cherry tomatoes, quartered
- 2 cups lettuce

For the dressing:

- 1 teaspoon mustard
- 1 teaspoon lemon juice
- 1 tablespoon olive oil
- 1 tablespoon apple cider vinegar, organic
- Salt and pepper - to taste

Directions:

1. Chop the ham in cubes and cook in non-stick skillet, with few drops of oil for 3-5 minutes.

2. Meanwhile, slice the eggs and torn salad in bite size pieces. Place the salad in a bowl and top with quartered tomatoes, blue cheese, avocado and eggs. Add cooked ham and place aside.

3. Whisk the dressing ingredients and pour over salad, toss to combine and serve.

NOTE: Low-carb and rich in veggies and healthy fats, this salad is simple and fast meal that may help with weight loss.

Nutrition Facts

Serving Size 238 g

Amount Per Serving

Calories 378	Calories from Fat 272

% Daily Value*

Total Fat 30.2g	47%
Saturated Fat 8.8g	44%
Trans Fat 0.0g	
Cholesterol 207mg	69%
Sodium 1006mg	42%
Potassium 588mg	17%
Total Carbohydrates 8.9g	3%
Dietary Fiber 4.5g	18%
Sugars 1.3g	
Protein 19.2g	

Vitamin A 8%	•	Vitamin C 18%
Calcium 12%	•	Iron 18%

Nutrition Grade B-

* Based on a 2000 calorie diet

Chorizo salad
Serves: 4

Ingredients:

- 4 oz. radicchio, torn into pieces or arugula

- 4 oz. escarole

- 1 cup sliced Picante Chorizo sausage

- 1 garlic clove, minced

- 3 tablespoons extra virgin olive oil

- ¾ cup red grapes, seedless and cut in half

- ½ cup thinly sliced celery hearts

- ½ tablespoon finely grated lemon zest

- 2 tablespoons lemon juice

- Fresh round salt and pepper

Directions:

1. Heat some oil in a large skillet and fry chorizo until nicely browned.

2. Meanwhile in a large bowl combine all remaining ingredients and when chorizo is fried add as well, toss to combine.

3. Serve in a small bowls.

Nutrition Facts

Serving Size 117 g

Amount Per Serving

Calories 151	Calories from Fat 111
	% Daily Value*
Total Fat 12.3g	19%
Saturated Fat 2.1g	11%
Trans Fat 0.0g	
Cholesterol 13mg	4%
Sodium 112mg	5%
Potassium 253mg	7%
Total Carbohydrates 6.6g	2%
Dietary Fiber 1.7g	7%
Sugars 3.9g	
Protein 5.5g	

Vitamin A 24%	•	Vitamin C 18%
Calcium 6%	•	Iron 5%

Nutrition Grade B-
* Based on a 2000 calorie diet

Zucchini-strawberry salad
Serves: 2

Time: 15 minutes

Ingredients:

- 2 cups zucchini, spirals

- 2 tablespoons pistachios, shelled and crushed

- 2 tablespoons goat cheese, crumbled

- 1 teaspoon basil, dried and crushed

- 2 strawberries, sliced

For the dressing:

- 4 tablespoons avocado oil

- 8 strawberries

- 4 tablespoons balsamic vinegar

- ¼ teaspoon garlic, minced

- Salt and pepper – to taste

Directions:

1. Combine spiral zucchinis, pistachios, goat cheese, basil and strawberries in a bowl.

2. In a mini food blender combine the dressing ingredients, pulse until blended through.

3. Pour the dressing over salad, toss to combine and serve.

NOTE: Thanks to avocado oil and low-carb ingredients, this salad is perfect solution for weight loss, since fatty acids from the avocado oil "melt" abdominal fat.

Nutrition Facts

Serving Size 222 g

Amount Per Serving	
Calories 81	Calories from Fat 35

	% Daily Value*
Total Fat 3.9g	6%
Saturated Fat 0.8g	4%
Trans Fat 0.0g	
Cholesterol 0mg	0%
Sodium 15mg	1%
Potassium 501mg	14%
Total Carbohydrates 10.4g	3%
Dietary Fiber 3.7g	15%
Sugars 5.1g	
Protein 2.1g	

Vitamin A 6%	•	Vitamin C 94%
Calcium 3%	•	Iron 5%

Nutrition Grade A

* Based on a 2000 calorie diet

Chicken and blackberry salad
Serves: 2

Time: 35 minutes + inactive time

Ingredients:

- 14oz. chicken breasts, grilled and shredded (you can also use leftovers)

- ½ cup artichoke hearts, canned, rinsed, drained and sliced

- 1.5oz. black olives, pitted

- 5oz. blackberries

- 1 tablespoon blackberry vinegar

- 7oz. lettuce

- 1 tablespoon extra-virgin olive oil

Directions:

1. Wash lettuce and place aside to dry, torn into bite size pieces and place in a bowl.

2. Drain and slice the artichoke hearts and spread over salad, followed by shredded chicken.

3. Add olives and raspberries. Drizzle all with blackberry vinegar and extra-virgin olive oil, toss to combine and serve.

NOTE: Chicken-blackberry salad is rich in flavor, will fill you up for longer time, but is low in Net carbs.

Nutrition Facts

Serving Size 426 g

Amount Per Serving	
Calories 490	Calories from Fat 200
	% Daily Value*
Total Fat 22.2g	34%
Saturated Fat 5.1g	25%
Trans Fat 0.0g	
Cholesterol 177mg	59%
Sodium 178mg	7%
Potassium 737mg	21%
Total Carbohydrates 12.3g	4%
Dietary Fiber 4.4g	18%
Sugars 6.5g	
Protein 58.9g	

Vitamin A 5%	•	Vitamin C 32%
Calcium 5%	•	Iron 31%

Nutrition Grade B+
* Based on a 2000 calorie diet

Sweet-pea warm salad
Serves: 4

Time: 20 minutes

Ingredients:

- 7oz.snap pea sugar pods, chopped into 5 slices per pod

- 1 tablespoon rosemary, fresh

- 4 tablespoon butter

- 1 tablespoon coconut oil

- ½ cup shredded coconut, unsweetened

- Salt and pepper – to taste

Directions:

1. Melt butter in skillet over medium-high heat. Add coconut oil and stir, add shredded coconut and stir until fully coated.

2. Add rosemary and stir until combined, lower heat to low and cook the coconut, stirring for 10 minutes.

3. Add the chopped pea pods and mix to combine. Cook for 5 minutes and serve warm.

NOTE: Crispy, hot, delicious and low-carb salad which may help you with weight loss.

Nutrition Facts

Serving Size 186 g

Amount Per Serving

Calories 439	Calories from Fat 347
	% Daily Value*
Total Fat 38.6g	59%
Saturated Fat 21.4g	107%
Trans Fat 0.0g	
Cholesterol 61mg	20%
Sodium 164mg	7%
Potassium 23mg	1%
Total Carbohydrates 5.0g	2%
Dietary Fiber 20.7g	83%
Sugars 1.0g	
Protein 16.1g	

Vitamin A 15%	•	Vitamin C 2%
Calcium 21%	•	Iron 25%

Nutrition Grade B
* Based on a 2000 calorie diet

Thai chicken salad

Serves: 4

Time: 30 minutes + inactive time

Ingredients:

- 1lb. chicken breasts, sliced into ¼-inch thick stripes
- 1 zucchini, sliced thinly into strips
- 1 red pepper, sliced thinly into sticks
- 1 ½ teaspoons curry paste, mild
- 3 tablespoons lime juice
- 2 garlic cloves, crushed
- Salt and pepper – to taste
- 1 bunch spring onion, chopped

For the dressing:

- 2 teaspoons agave syrup
- 2 tablespoons extra-virgin olive oil
- 2 tablespoons lime juice
- 1 tablespoon fish sauce
- 1 tablespoon chopped cilantro
- 2 garlic cloves, minced

Directions:

1. Combine curry paste, lime juice and garlic, season with salt and pepper. Place the chicken strips into bow and pour over curry paste, cover and marinate for 30 minutes.

2. After 30 minutes, remove chicken from marinade and grill on high for 5-6 minutes per side.

3. While the chicken is cooking prepare the dressing, in a food blender combine all dressing ingredients.

4. Combine prepared veggies with chicken and pour over prepared dressing. Toss to combine and serve.

NOTE: Fast and simple salad, rich in vitamins, high in fibers and low in carbs is great option if you want to fill up and lose some weight.

Nutrition Facts

Serving Size 214 g

Amount Per Serving

Calories 278   Calories from Fat 106

	% Daily Value*
Total Fat 11.7g	18%
Saturated Fat 2.0g	10%
Cholesterol 87mg	29%
Sodium 428mg	18%
Potassium 432mg	12%
Total Carbohydrates 7.9g	3%
Dietary Fiber 1.2g	5%
Sugars 2.3g	
Protein 34.3g	

Vitamin A 21%	•	Vitamin C 79%
Calcium 3%	•	Iron 8%

Nutrition Grade B+

* Based on a 2000 calorie diet

Tuna salad

Serves: 2

Time: 20 minutes

Ingredients:

- 2 cups mixed greens
- 1 green onion, sliced
- 1 avocado, sliced
- 7oz. tuna, can
- 1 tablespoon balsamic vinegar
- ¼ cup min, fresh, chopped
- 2 tomatoes, diced
- ½ cup olives, pitted and chopped
- ½ cup parsley, chopped
- 2 tablespoons extra-virgin olive oil
- 2 zucchinis, small, sliced thinly
- Salt and pepper – to taste

Directions:

1. Grill the zucchinis in grill pan until for few seconds per side. Remove from the pan, allow to cool ad cut into bite size pieces.
2. Add remaining ingredients and toss to combine.
3. Serve after.

NOTE: Salad is rich in dietary fiber, loaded with vitamins and will fill you up for longer time and suppress appetite.

Nutrition Facts

Serving Size 443 g

Amount Per Serving

Calories 551 | Calories from Fat 378

	% Daily Value*
Total Fat 42.0g	65%
Saturated Fat 7.8g	39%
Trans Fat 0.0g	
Cholesterol 31mg	10%
Sodium 106mg	4%
Potassium 1315mg	38%
Total Carbohydrates 16.9g	6%
Dietary Fiber 8.1g	32%
Sugars 2.1g	
Protein 31.2g	

Vitamin A 69%	•	Vitamin C 121%
Calcium 7%	•	Iron 19%

Nutrition Grade B+

* Based on a 2000 calorie diet

Meat based recipes

Spicy chicken wings
Serves: 6

Time: 45 minutes

Ingredients:

- 2lb. chicken wings

- 1 cup tomato puree

- 2 tablespoons poultry seasoning

- ½ cup sugar-free syrup

- 1 tablespoon hot sauce

- 1 cup water

- 1 ½ teaspoons garlic, chopped

- Salt and pepper – to taste

Directions:

1. Combine tomato puree, water, syrup, poultry seasoning and chopped garlic in large sauce pan. Bring to boil over medium-high heat.

2. Add wings to the pot and reduce heat simmer, covered for 5 minutes.

3. Uncover wings and simmer for 20 minutes more.

4. Transfer wings onto wide plate and continue simmering sauce for 5 minutes or until slightly thickens. Season sauce with salt and pepper, add hot sauce and return wings to the pot, stir to coat well. Meanwhile, preheat broiler.

5. Arrange wings onto broiler pan and cook for 5 minutes per side or until crispy. Serve while still hot.

NOTE: Hot sauce contains chili and is well known that chili acts like metabolism booster.

Nutrition Facts

Serving Size 385 g

Amount Per Serving

Calories 477   Calories from Fat 154

% Daily Value*

Total Fat 17.1g	26%
Saturated Fat 4.7g	24%
Cholesterol 202mg	67%
Sodium 340mg	14%
Potassium 848mg	24%
Total Carbohydrates 11.2g	4%
Dietary Fiber 1.4g	6%
Sugars 3.1g	
Protein 66.9g	

Vitamin A 10%	•	Vitamin C 16%
Calcium 7%	•	Iron 25%

Nutrition Grade B

* Based on a 2000 calorie diet

Bacon with veal liver and peppercorns
Serves: 4

Time: 25 minutes

Ingredients:

- 8 pieces bacon

- 1 ¼ lb. veal liver, cut into slices

- 2 tablespoons green peppercorns, whole

- ½ brown onion, sliced thinly

Directions:

1. Heat non-stick skillet over medium high heat.

2. Add bacon and cook until crispy. Place on paper towels to drain and crumble.

3. Place onions in same pan where bacon cooked. Cook onions until tender, for 5 minutes.

4. Add liver slices and cook for 2 minutes per side. Transfer liver and onions onto serving platter. Place peppercorns into heated skillet just until warmed through.

5. Spoon over liver and add crumbled bacon. Serve while still hot.

NOTE: Veal liver is low carb-product, great for weight loss and rich in nutrients.

Nutrition Facts

Serving Size 166 g

Amount Per Serving	
Calories 302	Calories from Fat 89
	% Daily Value*
Total Fat 9.9g	15%
Saturated Fat 3.2g	16%
Trans Fat 0.3g	
Cholesterol 548mg	183%
Sodium 284mg	12%
Potassium 600mg	17%
Total Carbohydrates 10.8g	4%
Dietary Fiber 1.1g	5%
Sugars 0.6g	
Protein 40.9g	
Vitamin A 740%	Vitamin C 4%
Calcium 3%	Iron 55%

Nutrition Grade A
* Based on a 2000 calorie diet

Keto chili
Serves: 6

Time: 90 minutes

Ingredients:

- 1lb. beef, minced
- 1lb. sirloin steaks, diced in 1-inch pieces
- 2.5oz tomato puree
- 2 tablespoons fish sauce
- 2 tablespoons coconut aminos
- 1 tablespoon chili powder
- 1 onion, chopped
- 2 tablespoons cocoa powder
- ¼ teaspoon cayenne pepper
- Salt and pepper - to taste
- 1 teaspoon smoked paprika
- 1 ¼ teaspoon cumin, ground
- 1 teaspoon oregano or basil, dried
- 4 garlic cloves, minced
- 3tablespoons ghee
- 1 ¼ cup beef broth
- 2 green bell peppers, chopped and seeded

Directions:

1. Grease pan with ghee and heat over medium-high heat, add garlic with onion and cook for 5-7 minutes, stirring.

2. Add sirloin and minced beef and cook until browned on all sides.

3. Combine all dry spices in small bowl, cumin, paprika, chili powder, cayenne, salt, pepper, cocoa and oregano. Combine the spice mix with tomato puree and pour over browned meat.

4. Stir in beef broth, coconut aminos and fish sauce, reduce heat to medium, cover and simmer for 45 minutes. Stir in green peppers and cook for 10 minutes more. Serve after.

NOTE: Hearty, low-carb and rich in protein are main characteristic of this chili. It will fill you up without bad carbs.

Nutrition Facts

Serving Size 290 g

Amount Per Serving

Calories 386	Calories from Fat 152

	% Daily Value*
Total Fat 16.9g	26%
Saturated Fat 7.8g	39%
Cholesterol 152mg	51%
Sodium 742mg	31%
Potassium 931mg	27%
Total Carbohydrates 8.5g	3%
Dietary Fiber 2.8g	11%
Sugars 3.6g	
Protein 48.7g	

Vitamin A 42%	•	Vitamin C 92%
Calcium 3%	•	Iron 167%

Nutrition Grade A-

* Based on a 2000 calorie diet

Beef Danish meatballs
Serves: 6

Time: 30 minutes

Ingredients:

- 1lb. beef, ground
- 1 egg
- 1 cup ricotta cheese
- 1 ½ teaspoons allspice
- 1 ½ teaspoons nutmeg
- 4oz. Swiss cheese
- 4oz. white onion, minced
- 1 tablespoon butter
- 1 ½ teaspoons salt
- Pinch of black pepper

Directions:

1. Melt butter in skillet over medium-high heat, add onions and cook until tender. Remove from the heat and cool for 10 minutes.

2. Shred the Swiss cheese and place in food processor, process until you get a fine crumble. Place aside.

3. In a mixing bowl, combine egg with ricotta cheese. Stir in spices and mix until blended thoroughly. Stir in onions and cheese and finally add beef. Mix until ingredients come together.

4. Preheat oven to 350F and line baking sheet with parchment paper. Form 30 meat balls from the mixture and place onto baking sheet. Bake the meatballs for 20 minutes, serve after with fresh salad

NOTE: These meatballs are delicious, soft and low-carb, which makes them perfect for weight loss and Keto diet.

Nutrition Facts

Serving Size 167 g

Amount Per Serving

Calories 308 | Calories from Fat 145

	% Daily Value*
Total Fat 16.1g	25%
Saturated Fat 8.8g	44%
Cholesterol 130mg	43%
Sodium 744mg	31%
Potassium 416mg	12%
Total Carbohydrates 5.6g	2%
Dietary Fiber 0.6g	2%
Sugars 1.4g	
Protein 33.9g	

Vitamin A 8%	•	Vitamin C 3%
Calcium 28%	•	Iron 81%

Nutrition Grade B

* Based on a 2000 calorie diet

Stuffed meatloaf
Serves: 6

Time: 70 minutes

Ingredients:

- 2lb. beef, ground
- 3 scallions, chopped
- 3 garlic cloves, minced
- 2 tablespoons tomato paste
- 2 eggs, whole
- 4oz. goat cheese
- Handful of spinach
- Salt and pepper – to taste
- 2 teaspoons basil, dried
- ½ tablespoon rosemary, fresh, chopped

Directions:

1. Preheat oven to 425F.

2. Combine meat with eggs and scallions in a bowl. Add salt, pepper, basil and rosemary and mix until blended thoroughly.

3. Place the meat onto piece of plastic wrap and cover with other plastic wrap, flatten the meat to ¼-inch thick rectangle. Place the cheese and spinach on one shorter end and roll the meat using plastic foil.

4. Transfer the prepared meatloaf into baking dish and cover with tomato puree.

5. Cook for 55-60 minutes and remove from the oven, cover with foil and let the meatloaf rest for 10 minutes, serve after.

NOTE: This delicious meatloaf is great thing to serve for dinner since it only has few carbs and therefore you can enjoy freely.

Nutrition Facts

Serving Size 200 g

Amount Per Serving

Calories 397 | Calories from Fat 159

% Daily Value*

Total Fat 17.7g	27%
Saturated Fat 8.7g	43%
Cholesterol 210mg	70%
Sodium 192mg	8%
Potassium 722mg	21%
Total Carbohydrates 2.8g	1%
Dietary Fiber 0.6g	2%
Sugars 1.4g	
Protein 54.0g	

Vitamin A 12%	Vitamin C 5%
Calcium 19%	Iron 164%

Nutrition Grade B+

* Based on a 2000 calorie diet

Slow cooker chicken fajitas

Serves: 4

Ingredients:

- 1 ½ lb. chicken breasts, boneless and skinless
- ½ teaspoon ground coriander
- 1 teaspoon cumin
- Fresh ground salt and pepper – to taste
- 1 white onion, chopped
- 1 tablespoon chopped garlic
- 1 teaspoon chili powder
- 15oz. tomatoes, peeled and pureed in food blender
- ½ cup shredded cheese – by your choice

Directions:

1. Place onion and garlic in bottom of slow cooker. Top with chicken.
2. Combine spices in bowl and sprinkle evenly over chicken.
3. Add remaining ingredients and cover the slow cooker.
4. Cook on high for 4-5 hours.
5. Remove chicken and slice before serving.
6. Serve with low-carb tortilla and sprinkle with shredded cheese.

NOTE: Thanks to slow cooker you can prepare your dinner in advance just pop all in slow cooker and let it do all the cooking, while you can exercise and at the end of day treat yourself with low-carb delicious meal.

Nutrition Facts

Serving Size 205 g

Amount Per Serving

Calories 240	Calories from Fat 78

% Daily Value*

Total Fat 8.7g	13%
Saturated Fat 2.3g	12%
Cholesterol 101mg	34%
Sodium 107mg	4%
Potassium 491mg	14%
Total Carbohydrates 5.3g	2%
Dietary Fiber 1.5g	6%
Sugars 2.7g	
Protein 33.8g	

Vitamin A 16%	Vitamin C 20%
Calcium 4%	Iron 11%

Nutrition Grade A-

* Based on a 2000 calorie diet

Creamy steak
Serves: 4

Time: 30 minutes

Ingredients:

- 4 slices Swiss cheese

- 1lb. steak, shaved

- 1 tablespoon mustard

- ¼ cup onions, chopped

- 1 tablespoon ghee

- ¼ cup green pepper, chopped

- 2 tablespoons mayonnaise

- 1 tablespoon olive oil

- 1 tablespoon garlic, minced

Directions:

1. Melt ghee over medium-low heat in a frying pan. Add in garlic, onion and pepper. Cook until tender, stirring for 5-6 minutes.

2. Add olive oil and shaved steak, cook the steak all the way through for 7-8 minutes.

3. Turn the heat to low and add mayonnaise and mustard, stir well and top the meat with cheese slices. Allow to stand for 1 minute or until melted.

4. Mix once again and serve after.

Nutrition Facts

Serving Size 174 g

Amount Per Serving	
Calories 439	Calories from Fat 211

	% Daily Value*
Total Fat 23.4g	36%
Saturated Fat 9.8g	49%
Cholesterol 138mg	46%
Sodium 158mg	7%
Potassium 449mg	13%
Total Carbohydrates 5.9g	2%
Dietary Fiber 0.7g	3%
Sugars 1.5g	
Protein 49.5g	

Vitamin A 7%	•	Vitamin C 10%
Calcium 25%	•	Iron 23%

Nutrition Grade B-

* Based on a 2000 calorie diet

Easy taco pie
Serves: 8

Time: 40 minutes

Ingredients:

- 1 lb. beef, ground
- 6 eggs
- 2 garlic cloves, minced
- Salt and pepper – to taste
- 1 cup heavy cream
- 1 cup Cheddar cheese, shredded
- ¾ cup water
- 3 tablespoon taco seasoning

Directions:

1. Preheat oven to 350F and grease 9-inch baking ceramic pan.

2. Brown beef in large skillet over medium-high heat. Add taco seasoning and stir, add water and reduce heat to medium-low. Cook for few minutes until sauce is thickened.

3. Spread beef in prepared pan and place aside. Whisk eggs with cream, salt, pepper and garlic. Pour over beef and top with cheese, bake for 30 minutes or until center is set. Serve topped with tomato or avocado.

NOTE: The Combination of meat and eggs will leave you feeling fuller for longer, so you will eat less, which is actually good for weight loss and since this dish is very low in carbs it is a real hit.

Nutrition Facts

Serving Size 284 g

Amount Per Serving

Calories 525	Calories from Fat 307

	% Daily Value*
Total Fat 34.1g	52%
Saturated Fat 17.6g	88%
Cholesterol 418mg	139%
Sodium 355mg	15%
Potassium 602mg	17%
Total Carbohydrates 2.2g	1%
Sugars 0.7g	
Protein 50.5g	

Vitamin A 21%	•	Vitamin C 1%
Calcium 26%	•	Iron 127%

Nutrition Grade B
* Based on a 2000 calorie diet

Seafood based recipes

Coconut shrimp

Serves: 4

Time: 20 minutes

Ingredients:

- 1lb. shrimps, deveined
- ¾ cup coconut, unsweetened and shredded finely
- 2 tablespoons vegetable oil – to fry
- 1 egg, whisked
- 2 teaspoons water
- ¾ teaspoon salt
- 1 pinch black pepper

Directions:

1. Peel and devein the shrimps,place aside in clean bowl and cover.
2. Beat the egg in small bowl with water until slightly frothy.
3. In separate bowl combine together coconut, salt and pepper.
4. Preheat large non-stick skillet over medium-high heat, add 1 tablespoon oil.
5. While oil is heating up, dip shrimps in egg and in coconut mixture, one at the time.
6. Fill the pan with half of the shrimps, cook shrimps for 3 minutes per side.
7. Transfer shrimps onto plate, lined with kitchen paper to drain, and heat up remaining oil before cooking remaining shrimps. Serve while still hot.

NOTE: Loaded with protein, vitamin B3 and zinc, shrimps are excellent carbohydrate-free food for anyone who want to get rid of excess weight.

Nutrition Facts

Serving Size 150 g

Amount Per Serving

Calories 265   Calories from Fat 135

% Daily Value*

Total Fat 15.0g	23%
Saturated Fat 5.9g	29%
Trans Fat 0.0g	
Cholesterol 280mg	93%
Sodium 733mg	31%
Potassium 260mg	7%
Total Carbohydrates 4.1g	1%
Dietary Fiber 1.4g	5%
Sugars 1.0g	
Protein 27.7g	

Vitamin A 8%	•	Vitamin C 2%
Calcium 11%	•	Iron 15%

Nutrition Grade B-

* Based on a 2000 calorie diet

Grilled red snapper

Serves: 4

Time: 20 minutes + inactive time

Ingredients:

- 2lb. red snapper fillets
- 1 tablespoon extra-virgin olive oil
- ¼ cup white wine, dry
- 1 tablespoon parsley, fresh, chopped
- 1 tablespoon basil, fresh, chopped
- 1 ½ tablespoons lemon juice
- ½ teaspoon chili powder
- Salt and pepper – to taste
- 4 tablespoons chive, chopped
- 1/3 lemon, cut into slices

Directions:

1. Prepare the marinade, in a medium bowl whisk together olive oil, chili powder, pepper, salt, lemon juice, salt, wine, parsley and basil.

2. Prepare the fish, place red snapper fillets in a baking pan and pour over marinade.

3. Place lemon slices all over fish and cover with clean foil.

4. Refrigerate fish for 1 hour. Preheat grill and coat grill rack with cooking spray.

5. Remove fish from marinade and place onto grill rack.

6. Cook fish for 15 minutes, covered with aluminum foil. Fish is done when flakes easily.

7. Serve while still hot, garnished with chives.

NOTE: Red snapper is low calorie and high protein food which can help you with losing extra weight and lowering your risk for heart disease.

Nutrition Facts

Serving Size 261 g

Amount Per Serving

Calories 338	Calories from Fat 68

% Daily Value*

Total Fat 7.6g	12%
Saturated Fat 1.4g	7%
Cholesterol 107mg	36%
Sodium 135mg	6%
Potassium 1235mg	35%
Total Carbohydrates 1.4g	0%
Protein 60.0g	

Vitamin A 12%	•	Vitamin C 20%
Calcium 10%	•	Iron 4%

Nutrition Grade C+

* Based on a 2000 calorie diet

Salmon stuffed avocado
Serves: 4

Time: 40 minutes

Ingredients:

- 4 small avocados

- 4 tablespoons lemon juice

- 2 tablespoons ghee, melted

- 14oz. salmon fillets

- 5oz. white onion, chopped

- 4oz. sour crème

- Salt and pepper – to taste

Directions:

1. Preheat oven to 400F and place salmon fillets on baking tray lined with parchment paper.

2. Drizzle the fillets with melted ghee and season to taste. Drizzle with 2 tablespoons lemon juice.

3. Bake salmon for 25 minutes or until flakes easily. Place aside to cool and flake salmon using fork. Transfer in a bowl and add onions, sour crème and remaining lemon juice. Scoop the avocado flesh, leaving nice ½-inch thick shell and cut the cooped flesh into small pieces, combine with salmon and fill the avocado shells with prepared mix. Sprinkle with some dill before serving.

NOTE: Salmon is well known by its many health benefits,it is low carb fish and great and valuable source of nutrients and omega 3-fatty acids, while avocado fatty acids can also spot-reduce abdominal fat.

Nutrition Facts

Serving Size 256 g

Amount Per Serving

Calories 454 | Calories from Fat 340

	% Daily Value*
Total Fat 37.8g	58%
Saturated Fat 7.9g	39%
Trans Fat 0.0g	
Cholesterol 60mg	20%
Sodium 53mg	2%
Potassium 796mg	23%
Total Carbohydrates 9.7g	3%
Dietary Fiber 5.6g	22%
Sugars 2.2g	
Protein 21.7g	

Vitamin A 8%	•	Vitamin C 28%
Calcium 5%	•	Iron 6%

Nutrition Grade C+

* Based on a 2000 calorie diet

Creamy shrimp with bacon
Serves: 4

Time: 20 minutes

Ingredients:

- 4oz. smoked salmon

- 4oz. shrimps, deveined

- ½ cup heavy cream

- 4 slices bacon, cut into 1-inch pieces

- 1 cup mushrooms, sliced

- Salt and pepper – to taste

Directions:

1. Heat non-stick skillet over medium heat, add bacon and cook until juts crispy.

2. Add mushrooms and cook for 5 minutes. Slice salmon into strips and add to mushrooms, cook for 2-3 minutes.

3. Ad shrimps, increase heat to high and cook for 2 minutes, stir in cream, season to taste and cook for 1 minute.

4. Serve immediately.

NOTE: Seafood products are great if you are trying to lose weight since they are low in carbs but rich in nutrients our body needs.

Nutrition Facts

Serving Size 108 g

Amount Per Serving	
Calories 225	Calories from Fat 137
	% Daily Value*
Total Fat 15.2g	23%
Saturated Fat 6.5g	32%
Trans Fat 0.0g	
Cholesterol 108mg	36%
Sodium 1082mg	45%
Potassium 272mg	8%
Total Carbohydrates 1.7g	1%
Protein 19.5g	

Vitamin A 7%	•	Vitamin C 1%	
Calcium 4%	•	Iron 6%	

Nutrition Grade D+
* Based on a 2000 calorie diet

Bacon wrapped scallops
Serves: 4

Time: 15 minutes

Ingredients:

- 1 tablespoon vegetable oil

- 12 scallops

- 12 bacon slices

- Salt and pepper – to taste

Directions:

1. Wash and pat dry scallops.

2. Wrap each bacon slice around scallop and secure with toothpick. Season with salt and pepper.

3. Heat vegetable oil in large skillet over medium heat, place wrapped scallops into heated oil and cook 2 ½ minutes per side. Serve immediately.

NOTE: Scallops contain high amount of amino acid called trytophan that has been shown to regulate and suppress appetite.

Nutrition Facts

Serving Size 123 g

Amount Per Serving	
Calories 170	Calories from Fat 51
	% Daily Value*
Total Fat 5.7g	9%
Saturated Fat 1.0g	5%
Cholesterol 56mg	19%
Sodium 265mg	11%
Potassium 290mg	8%
Total Carbohydrates 2.1g	1%
Protein 19.9g	
Vitamin A 1% •	Vitamin C 5%
Calcium 2% •	Iron 4%

Nutrition Grade B-
* Based on a 2000 calorie diet

Baked salmon in foil
Serves: 4

Time: 30 minutes

Ingredients:

- 1.25lb. salmon

- 2 tablespoons butter, cubed

- ¼ teaspoon Italian seasoning

- 2 tablespoons lemon juice

- Salt and pepper – to taste

- 2 garlic cloves, minced

- ¼ teaspoon red pepper flakes

Directions:

1. Preheat oven to 375F and prepare baking dish.

2. Combine lemon juice and garlic in sauce pan, heat over medium heat allowing lemon juice to reduce to 1 tablespoon. Add in 1 tablespoon butter and remove from the heat, stir until butter melts.

3. Repeat with second table of butter, heating if needed.

4. Place the salmon onto piece of aluminum foil, large enough to close into packet. Generously season salmon with salt and pepper and pour over butter mix, sprinkle with red pepper flakes and Italian seasoning. Fold the foil to create packet and transfer salmon onto baking tray. Bake for 15 minutes. After the time has run, open the packet and broil the salmon for 2-3 minutes. Serve immediately.

NOTE: Red pepper flakes have a mild effect on weight loss, but most importantly this type of dish is low-carb and easy to digest.

Nutrition Facts

Serving Size 158 g

Amount Per Serving

Calories 244	Calories from Fat 132
	% Daily Value*
Total Fat 14.7g	23%
Saturated Fat 5.0g	25%
Trans Fat 0.0g	
Cholesterol 78mg	26%
Sodium 105mg	4%
Potassium 564mg	16%
Total Carbohydrates 0.8g	0%
Protein 27.7g	

Vitamin A 7%	•	Vitamin C 7%
Calcium 6%	•	Iron 5%

Nutrition Grade C

* Based on a 2000 calorie diet

Soups

Cauliflower and turnip soup
Serves: 6

Time: 30 minutes

Ingredients:

- 1.5lb. cauliflower
- 7oz. turnip, peeled and diced
- 2 cups chicken stock
- 3 tablespoons ghee
- 1 onion, chopped
- 5oz. chorizo, chopped
- Salt – to taste

Directions:

1. Wash the cauliflower and cut into small florets, set aside.
2. Melt 2 tablespoons ghee in Dutch oven and add chopped onion, cook for 5 minutes. Stir in prepared cauliflower and cook for 5-6 minutes, stirring.
3. Stir in chicken stock and cover with lid, cook for 10 minutes.
4. Meanwhile, melt the remaining ghee and cook chorizo with turnips for 8-10 minutes.
5. Transfer half of the chorizo mixture into soup, remove soup from the heat and blend using immersion blender. Season to taste, serve in small bowls and top with reserved chorizo mix.

NOTE: Low in carb and definitely health for you…this soup will fill you up, it is rich in fibers and may help with weight loss.

Nutrition Facts

Serving Size 276 g

Amount Per Serving

Calories 212	Calories from Fat 142

	% Daily Value*
Total Fat 15.8g	24%
Saturated Fat 7.4g	37%
Cholesterol 37mg	12%
Sodium 603mg	25%
Potassium 533mg	15%
Total Carbohydrates 10.5g	4%
Dietary Fiber 3.8g	15%
Sugars 5.0g	
Protein 8.7g	

Vitamin A 4%	•	Vitamin C 101%
Calcium 5%	•	Iron 6%

Nutrition Grade B

* Based on a 2000 calorie diet

Super soup
Serves: 6

Time: 30 minutes

Ingredients:

- 14oz. cauliflower heat, cut into florets
- 5oz. watercress
- 7oz. spinach, thawed
- 4 cups chicken stock
- 1 cup coconut milk
- ¼ cup ghee
- Salt and pepper – to taste
- 1 onion, chopped
- 2 garlic cloves, crushed

Directions:

1. Grease Dutch oven with ghee, place over medium-high heat and add onion and garlic. Cook until browned and stir cauliflower florets. Cook for 5 minutes.

2. Add spinach and water cress and cook for 2 minutes or until just wilted, pour in vegetable stock and bring to boil.

3. Cook until cauliflower is crisp-tender and stir in the coconut milk.

4. Season with salt and pepper and remove from the heat, process the soup using immersion blender until creamy. Serve immediately.

NOTE: Since soup is made from super food ingredients like spinach and watercress it must be good for your health and may give wanted support in weight loss.

Nutrition Facts

Serving Size 353 g

Amount Per Serving

Calories 211   Calories from Fat 169

	% Daily Value*
Total Fat 18.8g	29%
Saturated Fat 13.9g	69%
Trans Fat 0.0g	
Cholesterol 22mg	7%
Sodium 577mg	24%
Potassium 573mg	16%
Total Carbohydrates 9.5g	3%
Dietary Fiber 4.0g	16%
Sugars 4.4g	
Protein 4.6g	

Vitamin A 75%	•	Vitamin C 92%
Calcium 8%	•	Iron 12%

Nutrition Grade B

* Based on a 2000 calorie diet

Jalapeno soup
Serves: 4

Time: 25 minutes

Ingredients:

- 4 jalapeno peppers

- 4 slices bacon, raw

- 2 tablespoons salsa

- 2 cups chicken stock

- ½ teaspoon garlic powder

- 4oz. cream cheese

- ½ cup heavy cream

- 1 cup Monterey Jack cheese, shredded

Directions:

1. Cook the bacon in non-stick skillet until crisp, remove, chop and place aside on paper towel.

2. In same pan add heavy cream, cream cheese and chicken stock, bring to simmer over medium heat and cook for few minutes, stirring.

3. Whisk in salsa Verde, chili powder and shredded cheese. Continue cooking until cheese is melted.

4. Meanwhile, wash the jalapenos until charred and soft, peel the skin, remove seeds and chop finely. Add to soup and cook for 5 minutes.

5. Season with salt and pepper and continue cooking until soup is thickened slightly. Remove from heat, serve in bowls and top with chopped bacon before serving.

NOTE: Jalapeno peppers contain strong enzymes that boost metabolism and accelerate fat burn.

Nutrition Facts

Serving Size 224 g

Amount Per Serving

Calories 270	Calories from Fat 220

% Daily Value*

Total Fat 24.5g	38%
Saturated Fat 15.2g	76%
Cholesterol 77mg	26%
Sodium 1039mg	43%
Potassium 145mg	4%
Total Carbohydrates 3.5g	1%
Dietary Fiber 0.7g	3%
Sugars 1.4g	
Protein 10.1g	

Vitamin A 24%	•	Vitamin C 4%
Calcium 26%	•	Iron 6%

Nutrition Grade C+

* Based on a 2000 calorie diet

Keto tomato bisque

Serves: 4

Time: 60 minutes

Ingredients:

- 28oz. tomatoes, peeled and pureed
- 1 cup heavy cream
- 1 onion, diced
- 1 teaspoon fresh ground pepper
- 4 cups chicken stock
- ½ cup grated Parmesan
- 1 bunch celery, chopped
- ½ cup basil, chopped
- 1 tablespoon olive oil
- Salt and pepper – to taste

Directions:

1. Heat olive oil in large pot over medium-high heat, add onion, with celery and cook until tender.

2. Pour chicken stock and tomatoes in the pot, bring mixture to simmer and season with salt and pepper. Simmer for 30 minutes.

3. Turn off heat and using immersion blender puree until smooth.

4. Stir in heavy cream, basil and Parmesan cheese.

5. Serve immediately.

Nutrition Facts

Serving Size 338 g

Amount Per Serving

Calories 128   Calories from Fat 94

% Daily Value*

Total Fat 10.4g	16%
Saturated Fat 5.1g	25%
Cholesterol 27mg	9%
Sodium 524mg	22%
Potassium 375mg	11%
Total Carbohydrates 8.2g	3%
Dietary Fiber 2.1g	8%
Sugars 4.8g	
Protein 2.3g	

Vitamin A 30%	•	Vitamin C 33%	
Calcium 5%	•	Iron 3%	

Nutrition Grade B-

* Based on a 2000 calorie diet

Chilled avocado soup
Serves: 4

Time: 15 minutes

Ingredients:

- 1 ½ cup pureed avocado

- 1 ½ cup vegetable broth

- 1 teaspoon cumin, ground

- 1 jalapeno pepper, seeded and chopped

- 1 ½ cups heavy cream

- Salt – to taste

Directions:

1. In a food blender combine all ingredients by order.

2. Pulse until smooth and blended thoroughly.

3. Serve immediately or you can reheat soup for few minutes over medium-high heat.

NOTE: This soup combines two fat burners – avocado and jalapeno pepper. With regular consumption you will see the results very soon.

Nutrition Facts

Serving Size 282 g

Amount Per Serving	
Calories 208	Calories from Fat 178
	% Daily Value*
Total Fat 19.7g	30%
Saturated Fat 4.1g	21%
Trans Fat 0.0g	
Cholesterol 0mg	0%
Sodium 12mg	1%
Potassium 506mg	14%
Total Carbohydrates 9.1g	3%
Dietary Fiber 6.9g	28%
Sugars 0.6g	
Protein 2.0g	

Vitamin A 4%	•	Vitamin C 19%	
Calcium 2%	•	Iron 5%	

Nutrition Grade B
* Based on a 2000 calorie diet

Mushroom and fennel soup
Serves: 4

Time: 60 minutes

Ingredients:

- 4 tablespoons butter

- 4 cups vegetable stock

- 1 cup leeks, sliced

- 20oz. heavy cream

- 8oz. mushrooms

- 1 cup fennel bulb, sliced

- Salt – to taste

Directions:

1. Bring stock to boil over medium-high heat and continue boiling until reduced by half.

2. Melt butter in large sauce pot over medium heat, add mushrooms and cook until browned.

3. Add fennel and leeks and season to taste, cook stirring until tender.

4. Add cream and bring to boil, continue cooking until reduced by half, stirring constantly to avoid bubbling. Add reduced stock and stir to combine, remove from the heat and puree using immersion blender. Serve after.

NOTE: Fennel is excellent for fighting obesity as it suppress the appetite and creates feeling of fullness and acts like a natural fat buster.

Nutrition Facts

Serving Size 357 g

Amount Per Serving

Calories 385	Calories from Fat 343
	% Daily Value*
Total Fat 38.1g	59%
Saturated Fat 23.6g	118%
Cholesterol 128mg	43%
Sodium 180mg	7%
Potassium 368mg	11%
Total Carbohydrates 9.5g	3%
Dietary Fiber 2.1g	9%
Sugars 2.6g	
Protein 4.3g	

Vitamin A 36%	•	Vitamin C 12%
Calcium 8%	•	Iron 13%

Nutrition Grade B.
* Based on a 2000 calorie diet

Zucchini soup
Serves: 4

Time: 40 minutes

Ingredients:

- 1 onion, medium, chopped
- ½ cup dill weed, chopped, fresh
- 2 tablespoons olive oil
- 4 cups chicken stock
- 1 chili pepper, small, seeded and chopped
- 2 zucchinis, medium, chopped in small cubes
- Salt and pepper – to taste

Directions:

1. Heat olive oil in medium sauce pan, add onion with pepper and cook until tender.
2. Add chicken stock, season to taste and bring to simmer, continue simmering for 10 minutes.
3. Add zucchinis and simmer until is tender. Remove from heat and stir in dill weed. Serve after.

NOTE: Zucchinis are known to reduce weight and therefor are great for diets which promote weight loss.

Nutrition Facts

Serving Size 376 g

Amount Per Serving

Calories 102	Calories from Fat 67
	% Daily Value*
Total Fat 7.5g	12%
Saturated Fat 1.1g	5%
Cholesterol 0mg	0%
Sodium 31mg	1%
Potassium 500mg	14%
Total Carbohydrates 9.3g	3%
Dietary Fiber 2.5g	10%
Sugars 2.9g	
Protein 2.7g	

Vitamin A 12%	•	Vitamin C 36%
Calcium 14%	•	Iron 19%

Nutrition Grade A
* Based on a 2000 calorie diet

Broccoli cheese soup
Serves: 4

Time: 20 minutes

Ingredients:

- 2 tablespoons butter

- 3 cup vegetable broth

- 8oz. cheddar cheese, shredded

- 4 cups broccoli florets

- 8oz. cream cheese

- 1 cup heavy cream

Directions:

1. Heat broth in sauce pot and bring to simmer, add broccoli and simmer until tender.

2. In separate pot heat the heavy cream, cheddar cheese and cream cheese with butter. Stir until melted and combined.

3. Once broccoli is tender remove half and puree remaining broccoli with immersion blender. Stir in prepared cheese mix and add removed broccoli, stir well to combine and serve after.

NOTE: Broccoli is high in dietary fiber, nutrients and vitamins and therefore great for weight loss.

Nutrition Facts

Serving Size 301 g

Amount Per Serving	
Calories 358	Calories from Fat 274
	% Daily Value*
Total Fat 30.4g	47%
Saturated Fat 18.9g	94%
Trans Fat 0.0g	
Cholesterol 91mg	30%
Sodium 777mg	32%
Potassium 379mg	11%
Total Carbohydrates 6.0g	2%
Dietary Fiber 1.6g	6%
Sugars 1.7g	
Protein 16.4g	

Vitamin A 28%	•	Vitamin C 90%	
Calcium 34%	•	Iron 8%	

Nutrition Grade C+
* Based on a 2000 calorie diet

Cabbage-ginger soup
Serves: 4

Ingredients:

- 2 cups chopped cabbage
- 4 cups chicken stock
- 1 ½-inch fresh ginger, grated
- 1 teaspoon coconut aminos

Directions:

1. Bring the chicken stock to boil over medium-high heat.
2. Add the cabbage and grated ginger.
3. Reduce the heat to low and simmer for 20-25 minutes or until the cabbage is tender.
4. Stir in the coconut aminos and serve while still hot.

NOTE: Cabbage soup is known to cut down excess pounds and when combined with ginger which speeds metabolism and eliminates toxins from the organism, we can say for sure that ginger-cabbage soup is wonder soup.

Nutrition Facts

Serving Size 280 g

Amount Per Serving

Calories 20	Calories from Fat 5

	% Daily Value*
Total Fat 0.6g	1%
Trans Fat 0.0g	
Cholesterol 0mg	0%
Sodium 771mg	32%
Potassium 74mg	2%
Total Carbohydrates 3.0g	1%
Dietary Fiber 0.9g	4%
Sugars 1.8g	
Protein 1.1g	

Vitamin A 1%	•	Vitamin C 21%
Calcium 3%	•	Iron 1%

Nutrition Grade A
* Based on a 2000 calorie diet

Final Thoughts

Nutrition and fitness experts from *WebMD* highly recommend you plan your day to lose weight. This is exactly what this Ketogenic Diet does for you. Change is tough and quite frankly reducing your carbs and boosting fats is going to be a shock to your system initially. A good one but still a shock nonetheless.

*If you commit your heart and soul to the Ketogenic Diet Rapid Weight Loss Plan you WILL lose up to a pound a day, or 30 pounds in thirty days, but ONLY if you commit!

You will not lose weight and make it stick if you don't have a plan, both short term and long term.

It really helps to have your meals planned and healthy low-carb, high-fat, and moderate protein snacks handy in a pinch. Your willpower is weak when your energy levels dip or you are just plain hungry.

Make the time to set out your exercise and eating plan at least the day before, and preferably a week in advance. This is going to increase your success rate. Take the sample meal ideas from this guide and build off them. Use the underlying fast weight loss eating strategy you have learned with this book to develop your fat blasting plan farther.

Losing fat is hard work and by switching up your typical balance of energy burn with the Ketogenic Diet, studies show you can lose up to 30 pounds in the first month! That's got to make you smile!

Make the time to understand the mechanics of this quick weight loss diet, commit to regular and effective high intensity interval training, and you **WILL** get skinny **FAST**! I'm not about to argue with science and neither should you.

It's time for you to make the changes you need to get healthy and happy in your skin. Now you've got the tools to reach your fat loss goals quickly and make them stick. Say **YES** and get started today. Promise you'll be happy you did!

Thank you for downloading this book!

I hope this book helps you jumpstart your fat loss journey. If you enjoyed this book, then I'd like to ask you for a favor, would you be kind enough to leave a review for this boo. It'd be greatly appreciated!

Thank you and good luck!

Henry Brooke